CLINICAL EXAMINATION

AT YOUR FINGERTIPS

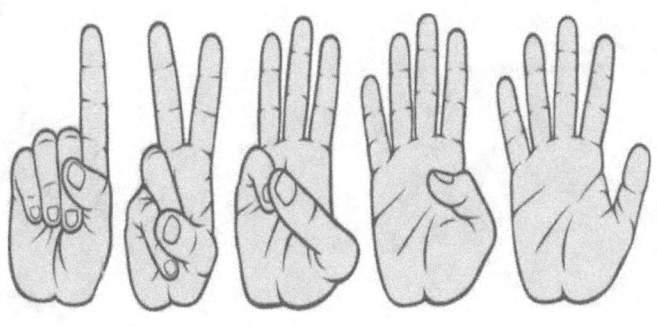

Dr Rao Maaz Bin Shakir
MBBS, MRCS (Ed)

INDEX

ABCDE

AIRWAY
-patient talking
-chin lift
-head tilt
-Jaw thrust
-Nasopharyngeal airway
-Oropharyngeal airway
-I-gel
-bag mask ventilation

BREATHING
-respiratory rate
-oxygen saturation

-central or peripheral cyanosis
-use of accessory muscles
-trachea central
-feel for chest expansion
-percussion note (dull/hyper-resonant)
-clear chest on auscultation (bilateral air entry/crackles)

-request ABG and CXR

-treat with high flow oxygen (15L/min) using non-rebreather mask

CIRCULATION
-pulse (normal/bradycardia/tachycardia) rate and rhythm
-capillary refill time
-peripheries (warm well perfused/cold clammy)
-blood pressure
-JVP (normal/raised)
-heart sounds (normal/muffled) and murmur

-request ECG

-treat with 2 wide bore IV cannulae and send off bloods including troponin. treat hypotension with fluids
-pass urinary catheter

DISABILITY
-capillary blood glucose
-GCS/ACVPU
-Pupils
-Drugs

EVERYTHING ELSE
-temperature
-rash/edema

ABDOMINAL EXAMINATION

(WINCER)
WASH HANDS
INTRODUCTION
NOTICE (check patient details)
CONSENT
EXPOSURE
-nipples to mid thigh. Preferrably exposed to underwear
REPOSITION
-lying flat

INSPECTION (foot end and then kneel down to look at level of abdomen from right side)
-shape of the abdomen (normal/distended/sunken)
    -distended 5F (fat/fluid/faeces/flatus/foetus)
-movements of abdominal wall (respiratory movements/visible peristalsis in intestinal obstruction/moving abdomen means no guarding)
-umbilicus
    -shape (circular and inverted/everted/slitted)
    -position (central/displaced upwards)
-pulsations (aortic for AAA)
-prominent veins like caput medusa
-scar marks or stoma (previous surgery also posteriorly)
-striae (white/pink/purple)
-pubic hair (convex/concave upwards)
-head off bed (to see divarification of rectus abdominis/hernia)
-hernial orifices on cough (epigastric/umbilical/paraumbilical/incisional/inguinal/femoral)

Ask about pain
Look at patients face
PALPATION
-light
    -gain confidence
    -tenderness
    -guarding/rigidity
    -temperature
    -superficial lumps/masses
-deep
    -tenderness
    -rebound tenderness
    -mass (sigmoid colon/mass RIF/hard feces/abdominal aorta/gastric mass/abdominal lymph nodes)
-palpation for viscera
    -liver   (distance   below   costal   margin   in cm/span/size/edge/surface/consistency/tenderness/pulsations)
    -gall bladder
    -spleen (3 methods) (you cant get above it and spleen is not ballotable)
    -kidneys
    -urinary bladder
    -AAA

PERCUSSION
-liver (extent beyond costal margin in cm)
-spleen (extent beyond costal margin in cm)
-urinary bladder
-for ascites
    -shifting dullness
    -fluid or percussion thrill

AUSCULTATION
-bowels sounds
    -rate (3-5/min)
    -intensity (normal intensity/increased/decreased)
    -frequency (hyperdynamic)
    -quality (tinkling)
-bruit
    -aortic (AAA)
    -hepatic (HCC)
    -renal (renal artery stenosis)

INGUINAL LYMPHADENOPATHY

MALE AND FEMALE GENITAL EXAMINATION

DIGITAL RECTAL EXAMINATION
-perianal pathology (skin tags/external hemorrhoids/perianal fistula/sinus)
-anal tone (normal/increased/decreased)
-anal fissure
-anal cushions (normal/dilated)
-active bleeding
-anal mucosa
-mass/hard feces/mucus
-finger stained (blood/fecal)
-prostate
-sacrum

GENERAL PHYSICAL EXAMINATION

THANKS
HELP PATIENT DRESS
WASH HANDS
SUMMARY
DD

BREAST EXAMINATION

(WINCER)
WASH HANDS
INTRODUCTION
NOTICE (check patient details)
CONSENT
-and chaperone
EXPOSURE
-waist upwards
REPOSITION
-lying at 45°
-hands behind their head
-hands pushing against their hips (pectoralis major)
-hands pushing against a wall (serratus anterior)
-leaning forwards over side of bed in case of large breasts

EXAMINE GOOD BREAST FIRST

INSPECTION (6S)
-site (periareolar (ductal papilloma))
-number
-size (<3cm or <5cm (fibroadenoma))
-shape (irregular (traumatic fat necrosis)) (discrete/well defined (fibroadenoma/phyllodes tumor))
-symmetry (carcinoma in higher breast)
-surface (bosselated (phyllodes tumour)
-scar
-surrounding and overlying skin (fungation/tethering/peau d' orange/lymphedema) (skin thickening/retraction (traumatic fat necrosis))
-colour (erythema (acute bacterial mastitis))
-nipple   8   D   (pagets disease/discharge/depression/deviation/displacement/destruction/discolouration/duplicatio n)

Also inspect inframammary fold

Ask about pain

PALPATION (TT SECC FFP TR)
-temperature
-tenderness (tender in acute bacterial mastitis/cysts and non tender in traumatic fat necrosis/breast carcinoma)
-surface (smooth in fibroadenoma/lumpy bumpy in fibrocystic changes/irregular in breast carcinoma)
-edges (regular in cysts/elongated in fibroadenoma/discrete edges in fibroadenoma)
-consistence (firm (traumatic fat necrosis/fibroadenoma/phyllodes tumor/cysts) hard in breast carcinoma)
-compressibility
-fluctuance (breast abscess/cyst)
-fixity (mobility in fibroadenoma/cysts)
  -to skin

-to muscles
-to chest wall
-pulsatility
-transluminability
-reducibility
-skin pinch test
-slip sign
-refilling sign

-inframammary fold palpation
-axillary tail of spence
-nipple discharge expression
  -ask patient to do it herself
  -if cannot then ask chaperone

COMPARE

REGIONAL LYMPH NODES
-normal side first
-axillary
-supraclavicular

In post mastectomy patients
-winging of scapula (long thoracic nerve damage)
-sensory loss in axilla (intercostobrachial nerve T2 damage)

GENERAL PHYSICAL EXAM
RESPIRATORY EXAM for metastases
ABDOMINAL EXAM for metastases
SPINAL EXAM spinal tenderness for metastases

THANKS
HELP PATIENT DRESS
WASH HANDS
SUMMARY

DDX
-cysts
-fibroadenomas
-fibrocystic masses
-breast carcinoma
-traumatic fat necrosis
-chronic breast abscess
-soft tissue sarcoma
-antibioma
-giant fibroadenoma
-duct ectasia
-cystosarcoma phyllodes
-lipomas
-granulomas
-epidermal inclusion cysts
-lactational adenomas

IX
-FBC
-ESR
-CRP
-CLOTTING SCREEN
-U&E
-LFT
-GROUP AND SAVE
-CXR
-ECG

-MAMMOGRAPHY/USG BREAST
-FNAC
-TRUCUT BIOPSY
-USG ABDOMEN AND PELVIS
-CT CHEST for mediastinal lymph nodes
-CA 15-3
-BONE SCAN
-MRI BREAST for differentiating scar from breast tissue/for breasts with implants/to evaluate axilla

CARDIOVASCULAR EXAMINATION

10 regions

(WINCER)
WASH HANDS
INTRODUCTION
NOTICE (check patient details)
CONSENT
EXPOSURE
-upper limbs/chest/abdomen
REPOSITION
-supine at 45°
-head supported by pillow

Ask patient if there is any pain
GENERAL
-look around bed for oxygen/medication/walking aids/observation charts/ECG

HANDS
-splinter hemorrhage/janeway lesions (infective endocarditis)
-tar staining
-capillary refill time
-clubbing
-peripheral cyanosis

-PULSE (RRV CCC)
-rate at radial pulse (72 beats/min)
-rhythm at radial pulse (regular/occasionally irregular/regularly irregular/irregularly irregular)
-volume (normal/high/low)
-character at brachial/carotid pulse (normal/slow rising in aortic stenosis/collapsing in aortic regurgitation/pulsus bisferiens/jerky pulse/pulsus paradoxus/pulsus alternans/pulsus bigeminus). Check collapsing pulse by lifting patient hand and first ask if he has shoulder pain
-comparison with other vessels (no radioradial/radiofemoral delay)
-condition of vessel wall (wall not palpable)

BP 120/80mm Hg (narrow pulse pressure in aortic stenosis/wide pulse pressure in aoritc regurgitation)

NECK
-JVP (raised >7-8cm of blood/not raised) by asking patient to turn left 30° and look for double pulsations that are not palpable.
-palpate carotid pulse

EYES
-mucous membranes (normal/pale in anemia)
-corneal arcus (old age/hyperlipidemia)
-xanthelasma

MOUTH
-oral hygiene
-central cyanosis
-roth spots (infective endocarditis)

FACE
-malar rash

EXAMINATION OF PRECORDIUM

INSPECTION
-chest deformity (normal shape)
-bulging
-scars (median sternotomy/thoracotomy/under left clavicle for defibrillator/pacemaker)
-pulsations
-prominent veins
-mass (pacemaker)

PALPATION
-apex beat
    -site (normally in 5th ICS mid-clavicular line/shifted)
    -character (normal/tapping/heaving)
-left parasternal heave
-palpable heart sounds
-palpable murmurs (thrill)
-palpable pericardial rub

PERCUSSION
-cardiac dullness (normal/increased)

AUSCULTATION
Put left thumb on carotid
-heart sounds (S1 S2)
    -intensity (normal/loud/soft)
    -splitting (absent/usual/fixed/reverse)
-added sounds
    -opening snap
    -ejection systolic clicks
    -mid systolic clicks
    -prosthetic valve i.e metallic heart sounds
        -one click corresponding to S1 (mitral valve replacement)
        -two clicks corresponding to S2 (aortic valve replacement)
-murmurs (IT CREEPS)
    -intensity (grade 1-6)
    -timing
        -systolic (pansystolic for MR with diaphragm on apex and axilla for radiation/ejection systolic for AS with diaphragm on right 2nd ICS parasternal edge then right carotid for radiation)
        -diastolic (mid diastolic for MS with bell on apex and left lateral position on expiration/early diastolic for AR with diaphragm on left parasternal edge 4th ICS with patient sit and lean forward on expiration)
    -character (rough/blowing)
    -radiation (axilla/shoulder/neck)

-effect of respiration (increased intensity on inspiration/expiration)
  -effect of posture (left lateral/leaning forward)
  -pitch (low/high)
  -site of maximum intensity (apex/tricuspid area)
-pericardial rub
-bruit (carotid/thyroid)

-lung bases for crackles of left ventricular failure

LEGS
-peripheral/pretibial edema (right ventricular failure)
-vein graft harvest scars

SKIN
-bruises (warfarin use)

THANKS
HELP PATIENT DRESS
WASH HANDS
SUMMARY

EAR EXAMINATION

(WINCER)
WASH HANDS
INTRODUCTION
NOTICE (check patient details)
CONSENT
EXPOSURE
REPOSITION
-move chair forward so you can move behind them

INSPECTION
-scars around pinna especially over mastoid bone
-skin changes
-ear discharge
-CSF otorrhoea
-battle sign
-bleeding

-inspect both ears and face for any obvious abnormality e.g facial palsy, scars

-otoscopy (wax/erythema/tympanic membrane perforation)

SPECIAL TESTS
-Wisper test (use tragus to close other ear, stand arm length away and wisper a number if not heard then half arm length and then close to ear)
-Rinne test 256Hz tuning fork
-Weber test
-Facial nerve
-Romberg test (stand with feet together then close eyes) (loses balance with eyes open - cerebellar dysfuction/loses balance with closed eyes - defective proprioception or sensory ataxia)
-heel toe walking

THANKS
HELP PATIENT DRESS
WASH HANDS
SUMMARY

ELBOW EXAMINATION

(WINCER)
WASH HANDS
INTRODUCTION
NOTICE (check patient details)
CONSENT
EXPOSURE
-shirt off
REPOSITION
-look at the joint with patients arm alongside their body in supination
-carrying angle (0-15° normal)
-patient standing

INSPECTION (SSS DESM)
-scars (arthroscopy ports/post operative)
-skin (psoriasis patches/gouty tophi/also check pinna for tophi)
-swelling (RA/OA/olecranon bursitis)
-symmetry (alignment of the elbow and arms)
-deformity (cubitus valgus due to malunion of lateral condyle fracture/cubitus varus due to
malunion of supracondylar fracture in children/ankylosis/flexion deformity)
-erythema (RA)
-sinus (post operative/infective)
-muscle wasting (previous trauma/neurological lesions or infection like TB)

PALPATION
Ask about pain
-temperature
-tenderness (lateral epicondylitis tennis elbow/medial epicondylitis golfers elbow/olecranon
bursitis students elbow)
-relation of bony prominences in an equilateral triangle (disrupted in dislocation)
-joint line (palpate head of radius in supination and pronation)
-rheumatoid nodules on extensor surfaces of arms/elbow joint
-ulner nerve hypersensitive in ulnar neuritis or tardy ulnar palsy/thickening in leprosy)
-antecubital fossa (brachial artery/median nerve/biceps tendon)

MOVEMENTS

Bring your hand to the mouth.

Bring your hand above head (if can hold, extensor mechanism intact) otherwise hand falls
to hit face.

actively, passively and against resistance
-ulnohumeral joint (extend and flex elbow)
-radioulnar joint (pronation and supination)
-locking (trauma/OA/osteochondritis dessicans)

REGIONAL LYMPHADENOPATHY
FULL SHOULDER AND WRIST EXAMINATION
DISTAL NEUROVASCULAR STATUS

THANKS
HELP PATIENT DRESS
WASH HANDS
SUMMARY

FOOT/ANKLE EXAMINATION

(WINCER)
WASH HANDS
INTRODUCTION
NOTICE (check patient details)
-patient shoes for pattern of wear
CONSENT
EXPOSURE
-underwear
REPOSITION
-initially standing
-then lying in bed

Gait
-normal heel strike/toe off gait
-each step of normal height (increased stepping in foot drop)
-smooth and symmetrical
-walk on tip toes (plantarflexors)
-walk on heels (dorsiflexors)
-stand on outside edges of feet (inverters)
-stand on inside edges of feet (everters)

INSPECTION (SSS DESM)
-3 arches
-look between toes for ulcer/corns/callosities
-look at plantar surface
-scars
-swelling
-symmetry
-deformity (previous fracture/ruptured achilles tendon/talipes/pes planus/hallux valgus/mallet toe/hammer toe/claw toes/overriding toes)
-erythema
-sinus
-muscle wasting

PALPATE
Ask about pain
-temperature
-pulses (dorsalis pedis/PTA)
-palpate achilles tendon (thickening/swelling)
-palpate joints/bones (tenderness/swelling/irregularities)
  -squeeze MTP joints
  -tarsal joint
  -ankle joint
  -medial lateral malleoli
  -distal fibula
-capillary refill

MOVE
-foot plantarflexion
-foot dorsiflexion
-foot inversion
-foot eversion

SPECIAL TEST
-simmonds/thompson test for ruptured achilles tendon
-tinel tarsal tunnel test

-anterior drawer
-posterior drawer
-talar tilt test

REGIONAL LYMPHADENOPATHY
EXAMINE KNEE JOINT
DISTAL NEUROVASCULAR STATUS

THANKS
HELP PATIENT DRESS
WASH HANDS
SUMMARY

GENERAL PHYSICAL EXAMINATION

5
-general appearance (well/mildly ill/very ill looking boy/girl/lady/man/old lady/old man
-physique (tall/short normal built/obese/wasted/emaciated/undernourished)
-posture and attitude (lying comfortably in bed)
-consciousness (alert/confused/drowsy/deeply unconscious)

-IV line/NG/foley/nasal prongs

VITAL SIGNS
-pulse 72/min
-bp 120/80 mm Hg
-temp (36-37 or 96.5-98.6)
-resp rate 20/min

JACKLETS
-jaundice (upper sclera/undersurface of tongue)
-pallor (nails/palm/lower conjunctiva/tongue)
-cyanosis (nails/tongue)
-clubbing (nails)
-koilonychia (nails) in iron deficiency anemia
-leuconychia (nails) in hypoalbuminemia
-splinter hemorrhages (nails)

FINGERS
-oslers nodes
-heberdon nodes
-bouchard nodes

HAND
-hand deformity
-hand size and shape
-tremor
-muscle wasting
-palmar sweating
-palmar erythema
-dupuytren's contracture
-hepatic asterixis (flapping tremors)

WRIST/ARM
-pulse
-excoriations (pruritis)
-needle marks (IVDU)
-tattoos
-bruising (clotting abnormality)

FACE

-pale conjunctiva
-yellow sclera
-corneal arcus (senile/chronic cholestasis/hypercholesterolemia)
-xanthelesma
-periorbital edema
-proptosis
-rash
-parotid gland

MOUTH
-glossitis (vitamin B12 deficiency)
-angular stomatitis (iron and vitamin B12 deficiency)
-aphthous ulcers (crohn's disease/behcet disease/HSV)
-pigmentation (peutz jegher syndrome/addison disease)
-telangiectasia (osler weber rendu syndrome)

NECK
-thyroid
-neck veins
-troisier's sign/virchow node (GI cancer)

CHEST
-gynaecomastia
-spider naevi (>5 abnormal)
-axillary hair loss

LYMPH NODES
-epitrochlear
-axillary
-inguinal

EDEMA
-ankle
-shin
-dorsal foot
-sacrum

DEHYDRATION
-tongue
-skin turgor
-sunken eyes

HIP EXAMINATION

(WINCER)
WASH HANDS
INTRODUCTION
NOTICE (check patient details)
CONSENT
EXPOSURE
-underwear with both hip joints fully exposed
REPOSITION
-initially standing
-lay patient supine for palpation

Gait- ask patient to walk a few steps and come back (antalgic/trendelenberg/waddling/lurching)
Walking aids- stick/frame/brace/shoes
Then trendelenberg test

INSPECTION (SSS DESM)
From front, back and sides
-scar (post operative anterior or posterior approach)
-swelling (soft tissue or bony)
-symmetry (ASIS and greater trochanter should lie in a horizontal plane)
-deformity (adduction/abduction/fixed flexion/leg length discrepency/rotational/lumbar lordosis/pelvic tilt)
-erythema
-sinus (TB)
-muscle wasting (gluteus/quadriceps)

Ask patient to lie down
PALPATION
Examine good side first
Ask about pain
-temperature
-tenderness
   -greater trochanter (trochanteric bursitis)
   -femoral head (deep to femoral artery at mid inguinal point)
   -adductor longus muscle (adductor strain/adductor contracture)
   -ischial tuberosity (turn patient to side)
-crepitus (OA by medial or lateral rotation)
-inguinal lymphadenopathy
-apparent leg length (umbilicus to medial malleolus -shorter in adduction deformity and longer in abduction)
-true leg length (ASIS to medial malleolus -fracture/perthes/OA/DDH) when measuring lengths, square pelvis by your elbow and hand on each hip

SPECIAL TESTS
-trendelenberg's test (positive if iliac crest falls on same side foot off for 30s shows weak

hip abductors on opposite side)
-thomas test (to unmask fixed flexion deformity -lumbar lordosis reappear on hip extension of one hip after bilateral full knee hip flexion)

MOVE (active passive and against resistance) crepitus
-flexion (thigh touch abdomen) 0-120°
-extension (prone or lateral. donot perform if thomas positive) 0-10°
-abduction 0-45°
-adduction 0-25°
-internal rotation (passive only) 0-30°
-external rotation (passive only) 0-45°

DISTAL NEUROVASCULAR EXAMINATION OF LOWER LIMB

EXAMINE JOINT ABOVE AND BELOW (SPINE AND KNEE)

THANKS
HELP PATIENT DRESS
WASH HANDS
SUMMARY

Ix
-FBC
-ESR
-CRP
-CLOTTING SCREEN
-U&E
-LFT
-Xray Hip and knee
-MRI hip (if required)

DDx
-OA
-RA
-pseudogout
-gout
-inflammatory/infective arthritis
-reactive arthritis

HAND EXAMINATION

6
(WINCER)
WASH HANDS
INTRODUCTION
NOTICE (check patient details)
CONSENT
EXPOSURE
-hands, wrists, elbows
REPOSITION
-position patient with hands on a pillow/table/lap with palms up

INSPECTION
-scars (carpal tunnel release surgery)
-swellings
-skin changes (erythema in cellulitis/palmar erythema, pallor in PVD/anemia)
-symmetry
-deformity [dupuytren's contracture/bouchards nodes/heberden nodes/swan neck deformity/Z-thumb deformity/subluxation of MCP/boutonnieres deformity/radial deviation of wrists/ulnar deviation of fingers)
-muscle wasting (thenar or hypothenar wasting/chronic joint pathology/MND)
-nail changes (nailfold vasculitis/pitting/onycholysis)
-elbows (psoriatic plaques/rheumatoid nodules)

PALPATION
-temperature
-capillary refill
-squeeze across MCP joints (tenderness)
-anatomical snuffbox (tenderness in scaphoid fracture)
-bimanually palpate MCP PIP DIP and wrists for tenderness
-elbows (psoriatic plaques/rheumatoid nodules)

MOVE
-finger extension
-finger flexion
-wrist extension
-wrist flexion
-FDP (flexion at DIP)
-FDS (flexion at PIP while holding other fingers)
-all thumb movements

-power grip (grip your fingers) (inability to make fist in carpal tunnel syndrome)
-pincer/precision grip (hold a pen or fasten a button on shirt)

RANGE OF MOTION
-prayer sign

-reverse prayer sign
-radial deviation
-ulnar deviation
-pronation/supination

PERIPHERAL NERVE EXAM
-MOTOR
   -median nerve (abduct thumb and resist pushing against it/weak opposition/weak OK sign in anterior interosseous syndrome)
   -ulnar nerve (abducts fingers and resist pushing them together)
   -radial nerve (cock wrists and resist pushing down)
-SENSORY
   -median nerve (over lateral border of index finger)
   -ulnar nerve (over medial border of hand)
   -radial nerve (over the base of thumb)

SPECIAL TESTS
-tinel's test for carpal tunnel syndrome (tap over median nerve at wrist reproduces symptoms)
-phalen's test for carpal tunnel syndrome (hold wrists in flexion together for 60s leading to burning/tingling/numbness over thumb)
-durkan's test/carpal tunnel compression test (press and hold in between thenar and hypothenar eminences with your thumb for 30-60sec will reproduce symptoms)
-finkelstein's test for de quervian tenosynovitis
-allen's test to asses ulner arterial supply to hand when radial artery is occluded (normal less then 5 seconds)

REGIONAL LYMPHADENOPATHY

FULL NEUROVASCULAR EXAMINATION OF UPPER LIMB

EXAMINE ELBOW JOINT

THANKS
HELP PATIENT DRESS
WASH HANDS
SUMMARY

Ix

-FBC
-ESR
-Rheumatoid factor
-Antinuclear antibody

INGUINOSCROTAL/SCROTAL EXAMINATION

4 special

(WINCER)
WASH HANDS
INTRODUCTION
NOTICE (check patient details)
CONSENT
-and chaperone
EXPOSURE
-umbilicus to feet
REPOSITION
-standing

INSPECTION 6S
Kneel at the side of the patient
-site
-size
-shape
-symmetry
-surface
-surrounding and overlying skin
-scar
-colour
-cough impulse

PALPATION (TT SEC FFP TR)
Ask about pain
-temperature
-tenderness
-surface
-edges
-consistence
-fixity
-fluctuance
-pulsatility
-transilluminability (place torch from posterior aspect of lump - hydrocele/epididimal cyst)
-cough impulse
-identify ASIS and pubic tubercle
-reducibility (ask patient to reduce themselve)
-get above the lump
    -can't (indirect inguinoscrotal hernia/congenital or infantile hydrocele)
    -true scrotal
-feel testicle
    -palpable with testis (hematocele/hydrocele/orchitis/torsion/tumour like seminoma or

teratoma/syphilitic gumma)
   -separately to testis (epididymal cyst/epididymitis/spermatocoele/varicocele)
-epididymis
-vas deferens

AUSCULTATION
-bowel sounds

COMPARE
REGIONAL LYMPHADENOPATHY
-superficial inguinal
ABDOMINAL EXAMINATION
DIGITAL RECTAL EXAMINATION

THANKS
HELP PATIENT DRESS
WASH HANDS
SUMMARY

DDX
INGUINOCROTAL
-inguinal hernia
-congenital/infantile hydrocele
-enlarged lymph nodes
   -infective
      -cellulitis of LL
      -venereal infections
         -syphilis
         -chancroid
         -herpes simplex
         -lymphogranuloma venereum
   -malignant
      -lymphomas
      -metastatic melanomas of LL
      -metastatic SCC of genitals
-undescended testis
-lipoma of the cord
-saphena varix
-femoral hernia
-psoas abscess
-femoral aneurysm

SCROTAL
-hematocele
-hydrocele
-orchitis
-torsion of testis
-testicular tumour

-epididymal cyst
-lipoma of the cord
-encysted hydrocele of cord
-lymphvarix

-torsion of hydatid of morgagni
-epididymitis
-spermatocoele
-varicocele
-hernia (inguinal/femoral)
-lymphadenopathy

Ix

FBC
-ESR
-CRP
-CLOTTING SCREEN
-GROUP AND SAVE
-U&E
-LFT
-CXR
-ECG
-scrotal ultrasound
-USG ABDOMEN AND PELVIS for BPH/post voidal residual volume/mass
-CT staging scan
-Tumour markers
  -AFP (yolk sac tumor)
  -beta HCG (choriocarcinoma, embryonal carcinoma, teratocarcinoma, seminoma)
  -ALP (seminoma)
  -LDH (seminoma)

INGUINAL HERNIA EXAMINATION

(WINCER)
WASH HANDS
INTRODUCTION
NOTICE (check patient details)
CONSENT
-and chaperone
EXPOSURE
-umbilicus to knees
REPOSITION
-standing

INSPECTION 6S
Kneel at the side of the patient
-site
-size
-shape
-symmetry
-surface
-surrounding and overlying skin
-scar
-colour
-cough impulse
-delineate anatomy
    -locate pubic tubercle

PALPATION (TT SEC FFP TR)
Ask about pain
Palpate normal side first then lump
-temperature
-tenderness
-surface
-edges
-consistence (soft elastic/doughy granular)
-fixity
-fluctuance
-pulsatility
-transilluminability
-cough impulse (hold root of scrotum with left thumb and index finger and ask to cough)
-get above swelling (hold root of scrotum with left thumb and index finger)
-feel testes (separate/not)
-reducibility
    -ask patient to reduce themselves, if not then use your flat palm to reduce yourself. If reducible, ask them to cough and see if lump reappears
    -first standing if not possible then lying

-occlude superficial ring then cough impulse
-deep ring occlusion test: occlude deep ring then cough impulse
-zieman technique (index finger on deep/middle on superficial/ring on saphenous opening then ask to cough)

PERCUSSION
-resonant (enterocele)
-dull (omentum)

AUSCULTATION
-bowel sounds

COMPARE
SCROTAL EXAMINATION
REGIONAL LYMPHADENOPATHY
-superficial inguinal
ABDOMINAL EXAMINATION
DIGITAL RECTAL EXAMINATION for BPH/malignant obstruction/chronic fissure

THANKS
HELP PATIENT DRESS
WASH HANDS
SUMMARY

DDX
-inguinal hernia
-undescended testis
-lipoma
-femoral hernia
-saphena varix
-psoas absces
-femoral artery aneurysm
-varicocele

DDX OF FEMORAL HERNIA
-inguinal hernia
-saphena varix
-cloquet node
-lipoma
-femoral aneurysm
-psoas abscess

IX
-FBC
-ESR
-CRP
-CLOTTING SCREEN
-GROUP AND SAVE
-U&E
-LFT
-CXR
-ECG
-USG ABDOMEN AND PELVIS for BPH/post voidal residual volume/mass

KNEE EXAMINATION

(WINCER)
WASH HANDS
INTRODUCTION
NOTICE (check patient details)
CONSENT
EXPOSURE
-underwear
REPOSITION
-inspection on standing
-palpation on lying supine on couch

Gait (normal/antalgic)
Walking aids (walking sticks/frames/crutches/brace/shoes)
INSPECTION (SSS DESM)
From front, sides and back by kneeling down infront of patient
-scars
    -anterior midline (TKR)
    -suprapatellar (quadriceps repair)
    -tibial tubercle (tubercle transfer for high riding patella/ACL surgery)
-swelling
    -anterior (effusion/synovitis/prepatellar bursa/infrapatellar bursa)
    -lateral (meniscal cyst)
    -posterior (baker cyst/popliteal aneurysm)
-symmetry
-deformity (valgus/varus)
-erythema
-sinus
-muscle wasting

PALPATION
Ask patient to lie down
Watch patient's face while palpating
Ask about pain
-temperature
-joint lines
-palpate the following with knee flexed to 90°
    -patella (borders for tenderness/effusion)
    -patellar tendon (tendinitis)
    -tibial tuberosity (osgood schlatter disease)
    -head of fibula (irregularities/tenderness)
    -medial and lateral femoral condyle
    -medial and lateral tibial condyle
    -medial and lateral joint lines (irregularities/tenderness)
    -collateral ligaments

-quadriceps
-popliteal fossa (baker cyst)
-straighten knee and palpate patella for crepitus
-continuity of extensor apparatus
-quadriceps circumference (compare 10cm above patella)
-effusion
  -large
    -patellar tap test
  -small
    -bulge test
    -cross fluctuation test
-synovial thickening (not possible to lift patella RA/TB synovitis)
-flexion deformity (fixed/correctable)

MOVE (active and passive) and feel for crepitus on patello femoral junction in trauma/OA
-flexion (-5 to 150°)
-straight leg raise
-lift leg from heel to see any hyperextension

SPECIAL TESTS
-posterior sag sign tested at 90° knee flexion (PCL rupture)
-quads active test (PCL rupture)
-anterior drawer test tested at 90° knee flexion (ACL rupture)
-posterior drawer test tested at 90° knee flexion (PCL rupture)
-lachman test tested at 20-30° knee flexion (ACL rupture)
-pivot shift test (ACL rupture)
-dial test (PLC injury)
-valgus stress test (MCL damage) (full extension if negative then in 30° flexion)
-varus stress test (LCL damage) (full extension if negative then in 30° flexion)
-mcmurray test (medial and lateral menisci)
-patella tests
  -friction test
  -zolen/clark test
  -apprehension test (displace patella laterally to see pain/anxiety which shows recurrent patella dislocation)

REGIONAL LYMPHADENOPATHY
EXAMINE JOINT ABOVE AND BELOW
COMPLETE NEUROVASCULAR EXAMINATION OF LOWER LIMB

THANKS
HELP PATIENT DRESS
WASH HANDS
SUMMARY

Ix
-weight bearing Xray knee (AP and lateral views)
-MRI knee

LUMP

(WINCER)
WASH HANDS
INTRODUCTION
NOTICE (check patient details)
CONSENT
EXPOSURE
REPOSITION
-Sitting on chair

INSPECTION (6S)
-Site
-Number
-Size
-Shape (spherical/ovoid/pear shaped/irregular)
-Symmetry
-Surrounding and overlying Skin (normal/inflammed/ulcerated)
-Scar
-Colour

-Visible pulsatility
-Cough impulse
-Pressure effects

PALPATION (TT SECC FFP TR)
-Temperature
-Tenderness

-Surface (smooth/irregular/lobular/nodular)
-Edge (well defined/ ill defined or diffuse/ regular/ irregular)
-Consistency (soft/cystic/firm/hard/bony hard)
-Compressibility
-Fixity (skin/muscle)
-Fluctuance (paget's sign)
-Pulsatility
-Transilluminability
-Reducibility

-Cough impulse
-Slip sign
-Sign of moulding/indentation

PERCUSSION
-fluid thrill

AUSCULTATION
-bruits
-bowel sounds

COMPARE
REGIONAL LYMPH NODES
DISTAL NEUROVASCULAR STATUS
UNDERLYING JOINT MOVEMENTS
GENERAL PHYSICAL EXAM

THANKS
HELP PATIENT DRESS
WASH HANDS
SUMMARY

DDx
-lipoma
-sebaceous cyst
-abscess
-soft tissue tumour
-bone tumour
-vascular malformation

NEUROLOGICAL EXAMINATION

HIGHER MENTAL FUNCTIONS (ABCD GROM)
-appearance (normal well groomed/unkept)
-behaviour (normal alert cooperative/restless agitated)
-conscious level (fully conscious/drowsy/confused/deeply comatose) GCS
Check GCS by first asking pt name and then where he is? Then ask him to open his eyes
and raise right arm/show tongue. If doesnot then elicit painful stimulus look for eye
opening and motor movements.
-dellusions and hallucinations (present/absent)
-general intelligence (normal)
-released reflexes (GGAPS)
    -grasping reflex
    -glabellar tap reflex
    -avoiding reflex
    -palmomental reflex
    -snout reflex
-orientation in time and place (well oriented)
-memory (good/poor)

SPEECH (normal/dysphasia/dysarthria which is disorder of articulation/dysphonia)
  - ask name
  - ask him to close eyes
  - ask him to describe the wall infront (wernicke)
  - touch chin, nose and ear (broca)
  - repeat "agar magar kyun"
  - complex q : do you wear socks over your shoes?
-dysarthria (alcohol/cerebellar disease/head injury/lesions of cranial nerves 5,7,9,10,12)
-dysphonia (disorder of phonation due to vocal organ impairment e.g vocal cords)
-dysphasia (disorder of language that may be expressive/receptive/mixed)

CRANIAL NERVES
-olfactory
    -smell with coffee/chocolate
-optic 5
    -visual acuity (snellen chart)
    -colour vision (ishihara plates)
    -field of vision (using red hat pin by confrontation method)
    -pupils (light reflexes direct indirect and swinging/accomodation)
    -fundoscopy (red reflex)
-occulomotor 5
    -ptosis
    -pupils
        -size (normal/dilated/constricted)
        -shape (regular/irregular)

- -light reflex (direct and indirect)
- -accomodation reflex
- -extra occular movements H manoeuvre (normal/double vision or restriction of eye movement/nystagmus)
- -trochlear
  - -EOM (medially and inferiorly)
- -trigeminal
  - -sensory
    - -touch , pain and temperature in 3 territories forehead cheek bones and jaw angles
    - -corneal and conjunctival reflexes
  - -motor
    - -ask patient to open mouth and if unilateral lesion then jaw deviates to side of lesion
    - -masseter, temporalis
    - -medial and lateral pterygoids
    - -jaw jerk
- -abducent (EOM laterally)
- -facial
  - -inspection
    - -facial asymmetry
    - -wide palpebral fissure
    - -flattened nasolabial fold
    - -inability to close eye
    - -dribbling of saliva
    - -absent wrinkling on forehead
  - -close eyes tightly (zygomatic branch)
  - -raise eyebrows (temporal branch)
  - -inflate cheeks (buccal branch)
  - -show teeth (angle of mouth deviates to normal side) (marginal mandibular branch)
  - -tense and flare neck muscles (cervical branch)
  - -loud sounds (hyperacusis)
  - -loss of taste (chorda tympani)
- -vestibulocochlear
  - -cochlear
    - -whisper test
    - -watch test
    - -tuning fork tests 512Hz
      - -rinne
      - -weber
      - -abc
    - -audiometry
  - -vestibular
    - -positional nystagmus
    - -oculocephalic reflex (dolls eyes) in comatose patient
- -glossopharyngeal
  - -sensory
    - -gag reflex
    - -palatal reflex
- -vagus
  - -speech (normal/nasal quality/hoarseness)
  - -soft palate (Ah test uvula moves away from side of lesion/position of uvula)
  - -ask the patient to cough (assess adduction of both vocal cords by vagus)

-posterior pharyngeal wall
  -Ah test
  -gag reflex
  -palatal reflex
-vocal cords
  -laryngoscopy
-accessory
  -shrugging against resistance (trapezius)
  -right and left turning movements of head against resistance (sternocleidomastoid)
-hypoglossal
  -tongue (size/shape/symmetry/wasting/fasciculations)
  -protrusion of tongue (deviates to side of the lesion)
  -tongue movements and power

SENSORY SYSTEM
-primary sensations
  -fine touch
  -vibration
  -position/proprioception and passive movements
  -sharp pain
  -temperature
  -deep pain
-cortical sensations
  -tactile localization
  -two point discrimination
  -stereognosis
  -graphesthesia
  -perceptual rivalry
  Check fine touch and pain at respective dermatomes starting from proximal end.

MOTOR SYSTEM
-bulk and nutrition (normal/wasting/hypertrophy) measure muscle circumference when in doubt
-tone of muscles (normal/increased/decreased)
  -For ul, shake forearm then check tone at wrist, elbow and shoulders.
  -For ll
    -leg roll (roll the patients leg and watch the foot flop independently of leg)
    -leg lift (briskly lift leg off bed at knee joint. Heel should remain in contact with the bed
    -check tone at ankle, knee and hip
    -ankle clonus (>5 rhythmical movements is abnormal)

-power of muscles (grades 0-5) in ul, ask pt to raise arm - at least grade 3, then check against resistance all powers if yes then 5 if reduced resistance then grade 4. If cant raise arm then ask for horizontal movements - grade 2, if not then give painful stimulus on forearm and look for flicker of movement - grade 1, if absent then grade 0. Check power by power grip, at wrist, elbow and shoulders. Similar in ll flex leg at knee if pt can hold it there then grade 3 if not grade repeat as in ul. Check power at big toe, ankle, knee and hips including abduction and adduction at hips and shoulders

-reflexes
  -superficial
    -plantar

        -abdominal
        -cremasteric
        -anal
        -corneal/conjunctival
    -deep
        -brachioradialis
        -biceps jerk
        -triceps jerk
        -knee jerk
        -ankle jerk
    -if absent do reinforcement if brisk check clonus
-coordination of movements
        -finger nose test
        -finger to finger test
        -heel knee test
        -tandem walking
-involuntary movements
        -tremor
        -tics
-gait (normal/spastic/high stepping/drunken/waddling/parkinsonism)

SIGNS OF MENINGEAL IRRITATION
-neck rigidity
-kernig's sign
-brudzinski's sign

CEREBELLAR SIGNS (DAD DR CHIP3S)
-dysdiadochokinesia (rapidly alternating movements)
-ataxia (finger nose test and finger to finger tests)
-dysarthria
-drunken gait (broad based staggering slow and unsteady)
-rebound phenomenon
-cerebellar nystagmus
-hypotonia
-intention tremors
-pendular knee jerk, past pointing, pronator drift (pronation or slow upward drift on ipsilateral side when outstretched arms palm facing up)
-scanning speech

Cerebellar signs (Methods) 3 plus 10
    - introduction, consent and ask name
    - gait broad based staggering gait (Drunken gait)
    - tandem walking
    - romberg sign (positive in sensory ataxia)
    - inspect posture for truncal ataxia
    - assess speech (Dysarthria and scanning speech-stacatto speech say british constitution and baby hippopotamus)
    - assess Cerebellar nystagmus (make H)
    - finger nose and finger finger tests (Ataxia)
    - spread arms (pronator drift) and touch my hand (Intention tremors and Past pointing)
    - push down on outstretched arms and eyes closed (Rebound phenomenon)
    - check in upper limbs (Hypotonia)
    - repeated hand movements (Dysdiadochokinesia)

- Pendular knee jerk (in sitting position)
- heal shin test

ORTHOPAEDIC NECK EXAMINATION

(WINCER)
WASH HANDS
INTRODUCTION
NOTICE (check patient details)
CONSENT
EXPOSURE
-below clavicles
REPOSITION
-sitting on chair

INSPECTION (SSS DESM)
front,back and sides
-scars (post operative/post infective)
-swellings (soft tissue/bony mass/thyroid/supraclavicular fossae for pancoast tumor)
-symmetry (torticollis)
-deformity (kyphosis/vertebral collapse/klippel feil syndrome)
-erythema (inflammation)
-sinus (post operative/infective)
-muscle wasting (previous trauma/neurological/infection e.g TB)

PALPATION
Ask about pain
Feel vertebrae/sides/front of neck including supraclavicular fossae
-temperature
-tenderness (midline/paraspinal muscles/cervical spondylosis)
-stepping
-mass (soft tissue/bony/thyroid)
-cervical rib
-feel for crepitus

MOVE
-flexion (touch chin to chest)
-extension (plane of nose and forehead horizontal)
-lateral flexion (touch ear to shoulder/decreased in spondylosis)
-rotation

Repeat movements with downward pressure on neck

TESTS FOR THORACIC OUTLET SYNDROME

-hand ischemia (cold/discolouration/trophic changes)
-Roo test
-Adson test

ASCULATION
-subclavian artery murmur

CERVICAL LYMPHADENOPATHY
DISTAL NEUROVASCULAR STATUS
-pulses
-dermatomes
-myotomes

THANKS
HELP PATIENT DRESS
WASH HANDS
SUMMARY

PAROTID SWELLING

Special 4

(WINCER)
WASH HANDS
INTRODUCTION
NOTICE (check patient details)
CONSENT
EXPOSURE
REPOSITION
-sitting on chair

INSPECTION (8S)
-site (below and behind lobe of ear)
-size (lemon sized)
-shape (globular)
-surface (smooth/lobular)
-surroundings
-skin (fistula)
-scar (previous operation/parotid fistula)
-symmetry
-colour (erythema in parotid abscess)
-texture (brawny edematous in parotid abscess)

PALPATION (TT SECC FFP TR)
Examine from behind
-temperature (hot in parotid abscess)
-tenderness (parotid abscess)
-surface
-edges (defined/indistinct)
-consistence (soft/rubbery/firm/hard/stony hard)
-compressibility
-fluctuation (cystic/soft/solid)
-fixity (to massetter checked by clenching of teeth)
-pulsatility (transmitted)
-transilluminity (cystic/solid)
-mobility (in how many directions)
-skin pinch test +
-slip sign -
-refilling sign -

-bimanual examination for deep lobe palpation and stones

PERCUSSION
AUSCULTATION

PAROTID DUCT EXAMINATION
opposite upper second molar tooth
-stone
-redness/edema/pus in parotitis
-palpate the opening and try to milk any pus present
-bimanual examination

COMPARE

REGIONAL LYMPH NODES
-preauricular
-submandibular

FACIAL NERVE EXAMINATION
-inspection
    -facial asymmetry
    -loss of nasolabial fold on affected side
    -loss of furrows over forehead
    -raise eyebrows?
    -wide palpebral fissure
    -drooling saliva
    -angle of mouth deviated to normal side
    -inflate and blow mouth
    -whistle
    -ask to wrinkle/raise eyebrows
    -shut eyes against resistance
    -show teeth
    -tense and flare neck

MOVEMENTS AT JOINTS
-movements of jaw restricted if malignancy involves TMJ

FULL ENT EXAMINATION

THANKS
HELP PATIENT DRESS
WASH HANDS
SUMMARY

DDX

UNILATERAL
-duct obstruction
    -salivary calculus
    -external duct compression
-infective
    -mumps

- parotitis
- tumour
  - benign
    - pleomorphic adenoma
    - warthin's tumor
  - malignant
    - mucoepidermoid carcinoma
    - adenoid cystic carcinoma
    - adenocarcinoma
    - lymphoma

BILATERAL
- LOCAL DISEASE
  - mumps
  - parotitis
  - sialectasis
  - sjogren's syndrome
  - neoplasia
- SYSTEMIC DISEASE
  - mikulicz's syndrome
  - sarcoidosis
  - tuberculosis
  - alcoholism
  - myxoedema
  - cushing's disease
  - diabetes/insulin resistance
  - liver cirrhosis
  - gout
  - bulimia nervosa
  - drugs
    - thiouracil
    - isoprenaline
    - phenylbutazone
    - high estrogen OCPs
  - severe dehydration
  - malnutrition

PERIPHERAL ARTERIAL EXAMINATION

(WINCER)
WASH HANDS
INTRODUCTION
NOTICE (check patient details)
CONSENT
EXPOSURE
-shirt off and legs exposed
-limbs/chest/abdomen
REPOSITION
-lying on bed supine
-pillow under head

Ask patient if they are comfortable or if there is any pain

GENERAL
-look for walking aids/oxygen/medication and examine patient from end of the bed

INSPECTION (SNUGGS)
-skin
    -hands (tar staining/wasting of small muscles of hand in thoracic outlet syndrome/tendon xanthomata)
    -face (xanthalasma/corneal arcus)
    -abdomen (scars/pulsatile mass)
    -legs (colour pale/cyanosed/red/discolouration due to hemosiderin/thin shiny skin/hair loss/lipodermatosclerosis/venous eczema/atrophy blanche/edema/muscle wasting)
-nails (tar staining/onycholysis/thick and brittle/nail fold infarcts/splinter hemorrhages)
-ulcers (malleoli and pressure areas)
-guttering and gangrene (venous guttering/gangrene/tissue loss). Look for gangrene especially between toes
-scars (amputations/amputated digits or leg/scars from vein harvesting/bypass procedures)

4 PALPATION (PC BOAT)
Ask about pain
Good side first

Temperature

-pulses (radial/brachial/carotid/AAA/femoral/popliteal/DP/TP any aneurysms/radiofemoral delay) first radial pulse for rate and rhythm and radio radial delay then brachial and

carotid (one at a time)
-BP on upper limb
-palpate abdomen with two flat palms above umbilicus for pulsatile mass (abdominal aortic aneurysm)
-right and left femoral pulses and radio femoral delay
-popliteal pulses with knee slightly flexed
-DP and PT pulses bilaterally
-temperature (proximal to distal on limb) with back of hand
-capillary refill (upper and lower limbs 2-3s normal) in a toe on each side then compare with central capillary refill time over sternum
-oedema (DVT/lymphoedema/post surgical)
-allen's test

AUSCULTATION (CALF)
-bruits (carotid/aorta/iliac/femoral)

BUERGER'S ANGLE AND TEST
-elevate each leg separately to measure angle at which it turns pale/white (<20 in severe PAD). This angle is buerger angle. In normal person toes remain pink even at 90°.
-Keep both legs elevated at 45° for 2-3 minutes. Then ask patient to hang leg off bed to see reactive hyperemia as it turns dusky purple. Buerger's test is positive when there is more than 1 to 2 minutes required for cyanosis or redness to appear.

DOPPLER EXAMINATION
-dorsalis pedis and posterior tibial (listen for triphasic normal/biphasic normal/monophasic waveform in PAD) by applying gel and placing probe on pulse

ABPI
-note systolic pressure (when pulse disappears) bilaterally for brachial/DP/PT using US probe (normal 0.9-1/ 0.4-0.7 in intermittent claudication/ <0.4 in critical ischemia/ >1 in calcified arteries in diabetes)

VARICOSE VEIN EXAMINATION (can have mixed arterial and venous disease) VENOUS SYSTEM EXAMINATION in legs

FULL CARDIOVASCULAR EXAMINATION and ECG and arrange for arterial duplex/angiogram

NEUROLOGICAL EXAMINATION (diabetic neuropathy)

ABDOMINAL EXAMINATION for AAA

THANKS
HELP PATIENT DRESS
WASH HANDS
SUMMARY

IX
-FBC
-ESR
-U&E
-SERUM CREATININE
-LIPID PROFILE

-HBA1C
-COAGULATION PROFILE
-ECG
-ECHOCARDIOGRAPHY
-COLOUR DOPPLER
-ARTERIAL DUPLEX
-CATHETER ANGIOGRAPHY
-DIGITAL SUBTRACTION ANGIOGRAPHY
-CT ANGIOGRAPHY
-MR ANGIOGRAPHY

PERIPHERAL NEUROLOGICAL EXAMINATION OF LOWER LIMBS

(WINCER)
WASH HANDS
INTRODUCTION
NOTICE (check patient details)
-comfortable/agitated
CONSENT
EXPOSURE
-expose waist down with underwear on
REPOSITION
-walk
-then lie in bed supine

GAIT
-ask patient to walk
  -normal
  -antalgic (reduced stance phase on painful side)
  -circumduction (stiff leg swung in arc due to contralateral pyramidal tract lesion)
  -shuffling (parkinsonism)
  -festinant (parkinsonism)
  -wide based (cerebellar lesion)
  -high stepping (dorsal column loss/peripheral neuropathy)
  -scissor (bilateral upper motor neuron lesion/cerebral palsy)
  -trendelenburg/lurching (unilateral hip abductors weakness like superior gluteal nerve lesion)
  -waddling (bilateral proximal muscle weakness like proximal myopathy)
  -ataxic/staggering/drunken (cerebellar lesion/alcohol intoxication)
-ask patient to raise up onto toes (unable to do if lesion of S1/S2)

INSPECTION
-muscle wasting
-fasciculations (lower motor neuron lesion)
-deformity

ToPCaRS

TONE
Ask if patient has any pain
Look at patient face while examining

-passively flex and extend limb while also internally and externally rotating
-let leg go straight, hold by knee and rotate it side to side
-put hand behind knee and raise it quickly, heel should remain in contact with bed (if raises it indicates spasticity of the limb)

POWER
-ask patient to raise one leg at a time straight off bed (if shooting pain reproduced beyond 45°, it indicates sciatic nerve impingement (Lasegue's test positive) as sciatic nerve is stretched
-ask patient to hold position against your movement (isometric) or actively resist you (dynamic). All joint movements including hip/knee/ankle/big toe flexion and extension as minimum
-grades
  -0 (no movement)
  -1 (flicker of contraction)
  -2 (movement if gravity excluded)
  -3 (movement against gravity)
  -4 (moderate power against resistance)
  -5 (normal power)

COORDINATION
-heel shin test (stroke one heel along other shin above down at least twice)

REFLEXES
-knee reflex (tap patellar tendon with knee slightly flexed by other hand) L3/L4
-ankle reflex (tap achilles tendon with hip externally rotated, knee flexed, ankle dorsiflexed) L5/S1
-plantar reflex (extension of toes first means positive babinski sign i.e UMN lesion)
If deep reflexes are absent, ask patient to hook fingers together as reinforcement/distraction technique called Jendrassik maneuver
-grades
  - + (hyporeflexic)
  - ++ (normal)
  - +++ (hyperreflexic)

SENSATION
-dorsal column
  -light touch (touch with cotton wisp)
  -proprioception (move most distal joint up and down)
  -vibration (128Hz tuning fork at bony prominences starting 1st MTP joint)
-spinothalamic
  -temperature (hot and cold tubes)
  -sharp pain (neurotip to distinguish sharp and dull ends)
Test one modality at a time in each dermatomal distribution L1 to S2

EXAMINE ANAL TONE/SENSATION/REFLEXES for saddle anesthesia
-reduced perineal sensation (cauda equina syndrome)
-reduced anal tone (cauda equina syndrome)
-absent anal reflex (cauda equina syndrome)

PERFORM BLADDER SCAN for urinary retention (cauda equina syndrome)

review basic observations

EXAMINE UPPER LIMB NEUROLOGY AND CRANIAL NERVES

FULL SPINE EXAMINATION

THANKS
HELP PATIENT DRESS
WASH HANDS
SUMMARY

RESPIRATORY EXAMINATION

(WINCER)
WASH HANDS
INTRODUCTION
NOTICE (check patient details)
CONSENT
EXPOSURE
-limbs/chest/abdomen exposed
REPOSITION
-supine at 45°
-head supported by pillow

GENERAL
-look around bed for oxygen/medication especially inhalers
-ask about pain
-look from end of bed to see if they are comfortable/in pain
-ask them to take a deep breath in and out and to cough for you

HANDS
-tar staining
-digital clubbing
-peripheral cyanosis
-radial pulse for rate/rhythm
-temperature
-tremor (beta 2 agonist use)
-asterexis (CO_2 retention)

MOUTH
-central cyanosis by lifting tongue
-angular stomatitis

NECK
-jvp at 45° (raised in cor pulmonale)

REGIONAL LYMPH NODES
-cervical

-supraclavicular

CHEST (FRONT AND BACK)
INSPECTION 8
-respiratory rate 20/min and oxygen saturation
-type of respiration (abdominothoracic/thoracoabdominal/thoracic/acidotic/cheyne stokes)
-shape of chest (normal/barrel shaped)
-deformity (pectus carinatum/pectus excavatum/localised bulging)
-pulsations
-prominent veins
-scar marks (sternotomy/thoracotomy/chest drain/pacemaker) by asking patient to sit up and hold hands out to check CO_2 retention flap and look at back for thoracotomy scars
-chest movements (depth of expansion/equal on both sides) by asking patient to take a deep breath in and out

PALPATION 6
-position of trachea (central/left/right)
-apex beat
    -site
    -character
-tenderness, crepitus
-vocal fremitus (increased/decreased) asking patient to say 99
-chest movements (reduced/abnormal) by placing both palms on upper chest and then over lower chest with thumbs in between
-chest expansion (normal >5cm)

PERCUSSION 4
-supraclavicular
-medial third of clavicle
-upper border of liver (5th ICS)
-percussion note (resonant/increased/decreased equal/unequal on both sides)

AUSCULTATION 2
Ask patient to take deep breaths in and out with their mouth
-air entry (normal/decreased)
-breath sounds
    -intensity/volume (normal/diminished or quiet)
    -character/quality (vesicular/bronchial/bronchovesicular)
-added sounds (ronchi/coarse and fine crepitations or crackles or rales/pleural rub)
-vocal resonance say 99 (equal/unequal)

Repeat above on back of the patient

THANKS
HELP PATIENT DRESS
WASH HANDS
SUMMARY

STOMA EXAMINATION

(WINCER)
WASH HANDS
INTRODUCTION
NOTICE (check patient details)
CONSENT
-and chaperone
EXPOSURE
-to underwear
-stoma bag taken off
-ask for a nurse chaperone if female patient
-ensure adequate privacy
REPOSITION
-standing then lying flat with one pillow

GENERAL

INSPECTION (SOS LP COMB)
From the end of the bed and right side of the patient
-site (RLQ - colostomy/RIF - ileostomy or urostomy/LUQ - transverse loop colostomy/LIF)
-output (high/normal/low)
-spout/flush (spout present in ileostomy/flush to skin in colostomy)
-lumen (single-end stoma/double-loop stoma)
-perineum (scars and anus absent in APR) patency of anus
-complications (prolapse/retraction/stenosis/parastomal hernia ask patient to lift head off bed/skin excoriations or erythematous skin/electrolyte imbalance/hemorrhage/ischemia/gangrene/psychosexual disturbance)
-old scars (previous stoma in CD) and scars for underlying procedure
-mucosa (healthy pink/inflamed/necrotic ulcers)
-bag and contents (liquid stool-ileostomy/formed stool-colostomy/urine-ileal conduit/urostomy/nephrostomy)

PALPATION
Ask about pain
-digital stoma examination: lumen (patency/stenosis)
-transilluminate to assess mucosa for ulcerations

-parastomal hernia (cough impulse)
-stoma bag (1 piece/2 piece)

AUSCULTATION
-bowel sounds (presence and character)

Assess stoma position when standing and sitting
ABDOMINAL EXAMINATION

Reattach stoma bag
THANKS
HELP PATIENT DRESS
WASH HANDS
SUMMARY

SHOULDER EXAMINATION

(WINCER)
WASH HANDS
INTRODUCTION
NOTICE (check patient details)
CONSENT
EXPOSURE
-shirt off
REPOSITION
-ask patient to walk a few steps and turn around to see arm swing
-ask patient to stand

INSPECTION
-posture
-winging of scapula
Front, sides, back, superior joints, axillae (SSS DESM)
-scars (arthroscopy ports/post operative)
-swelling (joint effusions/dislocated SCJ or ACJ/ruptured biceps tendon)
-symmetry (alignment of shoulder joint/muscle contour/drooping)
-deformity (bony deformity/internal rotation/external rotation)
-erythema
-sinus (post operative/infective)
-muscle wasting

PALPATION
Ask about pain
-temperature
-palpate
    -glenohumeral joint anteriorly and posteriorly
    -bony landmarks (SCJ/clavicle/ACJ/acromion process/coracoid process/proximal
humerus/scapula)
    -muscle bulk (trapezius/deltoid/infraspinatus)
    -axilla (head of humerus/lumps/axillary lymphadenopathy)

MOVE
active, passive and against resistance with patient standing. Feel for crepitus on passive

movement
-flexion (150-180°)
-extension (45-60°)
-abduction (150-180°) assess for painful arc
-adduction (30-40°) by bringing arm to opposite shoulder
-internal rotation (40-70°) (hand behind back and reach up as high as possible)
-external rotation (90°) (elbow flexed 90° and put hands behind head)

MUSCLE POWER
against resistance
-supraspinatus
-deltoid
-infraspinatus and teres minor
-gerber test for subscapularis

SPECIAL TESTS
-wall press test
-rotator cuff
    -supraspinatus -empty can/thumbs down/jobe test (abduct arms with thumbs down, against downward resistance)
    -infraspinatus and teres minor - flex elbows 90° and resist external rotation
    -subscapularis - gerber's lift off test (lift hand from back against resistance when in internally rotated position)
-shoulder impingement/neer's test (stabilize scapula with right hand and then flex patients internally-rotated-arm fully to look for any pain)
-hawkin's test (flex shoulder 90° and elbow 90° then internally rotate to look for any pain)
-painful arc
-scarf test (place hand on opposite shoulder pain in AC joint ipsilaterally)
-shoulder apprehension-relocation test (abduct shoulder 90° and hold wrist to maximally externally rotate to see apprehension/pain on face. If dislocated, it is relocated by apply pressure backwards on head of humerus) shows recurrent dislocations/shoulder instability
-axillary nerve function
-sensations over lateral aspect of deltoid (regimental badge region)
-stability
    -anterior drawer
    -posterior drawer
    -sulcus test

REGIONAL LYMPHADENOPATHY
NECK AND ELBOW EXAMINATION
NEUROVASCULAR STATUS OF UPPER LIMBS

THANKS
HELP PATIENT DRESS
WASH HANDS
SUMMARY

Ix
-SHOULDER RADIOGRAPHS to see dislocation/subluxation/bankart lesion/hill sach lesion
-USS ROTATOR CUFF
-MRI SHOULDER
-CT SHOULDER to look for bone loss at glenoid edge

SPINE EXAMINATION

(WINCER)
WASH HANDS
INTRODUCTION
NOTICE (check patient details)
CONSENT
EXPOSURE
-to underwear
REPOSITION
-standing
-supine

-gait: walk away a few steps, turn around and come back
-walk on heels
-walk on toes
-walking aids like crutches

INSPECTION (SSS DESM)
front,back and sides
-scars (post operative e.g discectomy posterior midline/post infective/thoracotomy/spinal surgery)
-swellings (soft tissue/bony mass e.g gibbus in TB/fracture)
-symmetry of shoulders and posture of head and neck (torticollis)
-deformity (thoracic kyphosis/vertebral collapse/klippel feil syndrome/scoliosis may disappear with sitting if due to leg length discrepancy/cervical or lumbar lordosis)
-erythema (inflammation)
-sinus (post operative/infective)
-muscle wasting of paraspinal muscles (previous trauma/neurological/infection e.g TB)
-abnormal hairy patches/fat pad (spinal bifida)
-cafe au lait spots (neurofibromatosis)

-cervical spine
    -asymmetry in supraclavicular fossae
    -presence of torticollis (head is pulled to affected side and chin is tilted to opposite side)
-thoracolumbar spine

-assess thoracic curvature from side (increased convexity in kyphosis). Ask patient to bend forwards and try to touch toes (see change in posture that is mobility of thoracic spine)

-look for prominent vertebral spine (fracture/tuberculosis)

-note lumbar curvature (flattening of normal lumbar lordosis in prolapsed intervertebral disc/OA/infections/ankylosing spondylitis) (increased curvature in women/spondylolisthesis/secondary to increased thoracic curvature or flexion deformity of the hips)

-simian stance (flexion of spine/hips/knees) in spinal stenosis

-lateral curvature (scoliosis) most commonly protective due to prolapsed intervertebral disc. Note whether shoulder/hips level. Check mobility of scoliosis by sitting up and bending forwards

PALPATION
Ask about pain

Palpate vertebrae spinous processes in midline occiput distally and lateral aspect of vertebrae for masses/tenderness and sacroiliac joints/sides/front (mechanical joint pain/joint infection)

Palpate supraclavicular fossae for prominence of cervical rib/tumour masses/enlarged cervical lymph nodes

Palpate anterior structures of neck including thyroid gland

-temperature

-tenderness (midline/paraspinal muscles e.g. mechanical back pain or spasm as in IVD prolapse/sacroilitis e.g ankylosing spondylitis)

-stepping (spondylolisthesis/fracture/tumour). Slide down to sacrum looking for step deformity

-mass (soft tissue/bony)

-chest expansion (reduced in ankylosing spondylitis)

PERCUSSION
-percuss down spine (tender in infections/trauma/neoplasms)

MOVEMENTS
-cervical spine

　-flexion (touch chin to chest normally)

　-extension (plane of nose and forehead horizontal normally)

　-lateral flexion (almost touch ear to shoulder normally/decreased in spondylosis)

　-rotation (chin should normally fall just short of plane of shoulders. feel for crepitus at this stage (cervical spondylosis)

-thoracic

　-lateral rotation (sit on bed with arm folded across chest and turn upper body)

-lumbar

　-forward flexion (touch fingertips to toes. Normal 7cm from floor). Look for compensatory hip flexion

　-extension (lean back)

　-lateral flexion (slide hand on side of leg to assess how far hand can reach down ipsilateral thigh)

TESTS
-schober's test (for ankylosing spondylitis)

-lumbar disc prolapse/sciatic nerve root impingement

　-straight leg raise (with patient supine, ask patient to actively raise straight leg in air to greater than 45° (shooting pain in ipsilateral leg shows nerve root impingement)

-bragard's test SLR 80-90° (straight leg raise until lower back/buttock/thigh pain or paresthesia. then dorsiflex foot will worsen symptoms is called bragard's sign. Or ask patient to flex neck will cause pain is called neri sign)
-lasegue's test (following bragards test, foot dorsiflexed, flex knee until symptoms relieved then flex hip will worsen symptoms)
-reverse lasegue/femoral stretch test (for femoral nerve root impingement. positive test pain in thigh/inguinal region)
-pelvic compression (in sacroilitis)
-lhermitte's sign (radicular pain on neck flexion in spondylosis/prolapsed IVD)
-beevor's sign (umbilicus moves to the side on neck flexion while lying supine and hands under head in T6-T12 spinal cord injury)
-abdominal reflex (upper quadrant T6-T10 and lower quadrant T11-T12)

Topcars
-sensations
-motor system
-reflexes
-tone
-coordination
  -heel shin test

REGIONAL LYMPHADENOPATHY

FULL NEUROLOGICAL EXAMINATION including peripheral neurology -cauda equina (saddle anesthesia/loss of perianal sensation and anal tone)
-deep tendon reflexes
-extensor hallucis longus (weakness suggests L5 root pathology)

FULL VASCULAR EXAMINATION
-rule out AAA
-vascular status of upper and lower limbs

FULL CARDIORESPIRATORY SYSTEM EXAMINATION to look for kyphosis related complications like restriction in ventilation

THANKS
HELP PATIENT DRESS
WASH HANDS
SUMMARY

Ix
-posteroanterior and lateral xray of thoracic spine to look for bony abnormality like fracture/metastatic deposit
-blood tests for anemia/infection
-CT/MRI spine
-bone density scan to assess for osteoporosis

SUBMANDIBULAR SWELLING EXAMINATION

Special 3

(WINCER)
WASH HANDS
INTRODUCTION
NOTICE (check patient details)
CONSENT
EXPOSURE
REPOSITION
-Sitting on chair

INSPECTION (8S)
-site
-size
-shape
-surface
-symmetry
-skin
-scar
-surrounding
-colour
-texture

Ask about pain
PALPATION (TT SEC FFP TR)
Examine from behind
-temperature (with back of your hand)
-tenderness
-surface
-edges
-consistence/compressibility

-fluctuance
-fixity/mobility (fixity to myelohyoid can be checked by asking patient to push their tongue against the roof of their mouth)
-pulsatility
-transillumibilty
-reducibility

PERCUSION
AUSCULTATION

WHARTON'S DUCT EXAMINATION
-use torch to look for erythema/pus/stone on either side of lingual frenulum
Wear gloves.
-palpate on either side of lingual frenulum to feel for intraductal stones/thickening of the duct
-BIMANUAL PALPATION OF SUBMANDIBULAR GLAND/SPACE/DUCT through the floor of mouth and massage submandibular gland to see clear saliva flowing into oral cavity. Submandibular glands are ballotable while parotid glands are not.

COMPARE

REGIONAL LYMPHADENOPATHY
-level 1 to 6 cervical lymph nodes

MARGINAL MANDIBULAR NERVE EXAMINATION
-show teeth
-inability to depress angle of mouth (malignant infiltration/previous surgery)
-facial asymmetry

HYPOGLOSSAL NERVE EXAMINATION
-deviation of tongue towards side of lesion on tongue protrusion (malignant infiltration/previous surgery)

LINGUAL NERVE EXAMINATION
-loss of sensation on anterior third of tongue (malignant infiltration/previous surgery)

EXAMINE CONTRALATERAL SIDE
PAROTID EXAMINATION
FULL ENT EXAMINATION

For sjogren syndrome, look for xerostomia and xerophthalmia (schimer test)

THANKS
HELP PATIENT DRESS
WASH HANDS
SUMMARY

DDx
-submandibular sialolithiasis/calculus
-dental infection
-inflammatory
    -submandibular lymphadenopathy/lymphadenitis
    -ludwig's angina

-neoplastic
    -submandibular neoplasm like pleomorphic adenoma
    -lymphoma
-developmental
    -ranula
    -plunging ranula
    -dermoid cyst
    -cystic hygroma
-sjogren syndrome

Ix
-plain radiography of floor of mouth
-sialography
-scintigraphy
-OPG
-FNA
-CT
-MRI

THYROID EXAMINATION

(WINCER)
WASH HANDS
INTRODUCTION
NOTICE (check patient details)
CONSENT
EXPOSURE
-neck and upper chest (shirt unbuttoned/off)
REPOSITION
-Sitting on chair with room for you to examine from behind

GENERAL INSPECTION
    -Demeanour (restless and anxious/docile)
    -Hair (Normal/brittle dry thin)
    -Face (wasting/myxedema coarse facies mask like facies)
    -Built (thin and underweight/obese and overweight)
-Hands
    -Fingertips (acropachy/normal)
    -Palms (warm moist and palmar erythema/cold dry rough and carpal tunnel syndrome)
    -Radial pulse for rate/rhythm (tachy irregular/brady) AF
    -Outstretched hands and place a paper (fine tremor/-)
-Eyes
    -Hyperthyroid (Graves)
     -Lid retraction (Dalrymple sign)
     -Lid lag (Von Graafe's sign)
     -Absent forehead wrinkles (Joffroy's sign)
     -Exophthalmos
     -Absence of convergence (Moebius sign)
     -Absent blinking (Stellwag's sign)
     -Naffziger's sign (eyeballs seen from above)
     -jellinek sign (increased pigmentation of eyelids)

-Hypothyroid
  -Periorbital puffiness
  -Sunken eyes
  -Loss of lateral third of eyebrows
-Hoarse voice
-Proximal myopathy (by abducting shoulders against resistance and by asking the patient to stand from sitting without using their arms and arms crossed)
-Pretibial myxedema (Graves)
-Delayed relaxation of ankle reflex (Woltman sign) in hypo while brisk in Graves

INSPECTION (6S)
Inspection of whole neck from front/sides/back
-Site (anterior triangle of neck)
-Size (butterfly shaped)
-Shape
-Surface
  -Colour
  -Texture (smooth/nodular/bosselated)
  -Overlying skin (redness/edema/scar/dilated neck veins)
-Symmetry
-Extent
-Pulsations
-Movement on degglutition (look up and swallow water)
-Movement on tongue protrusion (if swelling is small and midline) (look up and protrude tongue)
-Raise arms above head (Pamberton Sign for retrosternal goitre)

PALPATION (ask about pain and examine good side first) (TT SEC FFP TR)
-Behind (standard method first)
  -Surface (smooth/nodular/bosselated)
  -Consistency (soft/firm/hard)
  -Swallow water
  -Protrude tongue
  -Berry's sign (absent carotid due to malignancy)
-Front
  -Temperature
  -Tenderness
  -Confirm size, shape, consistency
  -Edges
  -Check lower extent and palpate trachea by asking for degglutition (retrosternal goitre)
  -Fixity to skin by skin pinch test and deeper fixity by contraction of sternomastoids and check mobility
  -Kocher's test (push goitre to one side leads to stridor due to malignant goitre or very large MNG making trachea scabbard)
  -Lahey's method to palpate each lobe if one lobe is more prominent
  -Crile's method for small nodules
  -Tracheal deviation (trial's sign is prominence of sternocleidomastoid on side of deviation of trachea)
  -carotid artery (berry sign in which malignant thyroid engulfs carotid sheath hence carotid pulse not felt)
  -miosis/anhydrosis/ptosis/enophthalmos (horner syndrome due to involvement of sympathetic chain)

PERCUSSION
-Percuss over sternum (dullness in retrosternal extension)

AUSCULTATION
-Auscultate over superior poles for bruit

RELEVANT EXAMINAION
-Palpate lymph nodes (submental/submandibular/pre auricular/post auricular/occipital/posterior cervical/anterior cervical/pre tracheal/supraclavicular)

CARDIOVASCULAR EXAMINATION for secondary thyrotoxicosis
ORAL CAVITY for lingual thyroid/macroglossia/tremor of tongue

THANKS
HELP PATIENT DRESS
WASH HANDS
SUMMARY

DDX OF SOLITARY THYROID NODULE
-colloid goitre
-thyroid adenoma
   -macrofollicular (colloid)
   -microfollicular
   -embryonal
   -hurthle cell
-dominant nodule of MNG
-cyst
-thyroid carcinoma
   -papillary
   -follicular
   -medullary
   -anaplastic
   -lymphoma
   -metastatic
-thyroiditis (hashimoto/riedel/de quervain)
-graves disease
-iodine deficiency
-developmental abnormalities

DDX OF GOITRE
-simple goitre
   -physiological
        -puberty
        -pregnancy
   -pathological
        -iodine deficiency/endemic goitre
        -simple diffuse goitre
        -simple multinodular goitre
-toxic goitre
   -graves disease
   -solitary toxic adenoma
   -toxic multinodular goitre (plummer's disease)
-inflammatory goitre

        -hashimoto thyroiditis
        -riedel thyroiditis
        -de quervain thyroiditis
    -thyroid cancer
        -papillary
        -follicular
        -medullary
        -anaplastic
        -lymphoma

IX
-FBC
-ESR
-CRP
-CLOTTING SCREEN
-U&E
-LFT
-CXR
-ECG

-TFT
-SERUM CALCIUM
-XRAY NECK AP AND LATERAL VIEWS
-IDL
-USG NECK for number of nodules/suspicion for cancer like calcification or vascularity/suspicious lymph nodes. To see microcalcification/hypoechogenicity of a solid nodule/intranodular hypervascularity which are features of malignancy. Also distinguishes cystic/solid/mixed nodule.
-THYROID SCAN
-FNAC
-SERUM TSI/THYROGLOBULIN

ULCER

(WINCER)
WASH HANDS
INTRODUCTION
NOTICE (check patient details)
CONSENT
EXPOSURE
REPOSITION
-Sitting on chair

INSPECTION (BEDS)
-Site (medial malleolus/nose/neck/heal/toe/sacrum)
-Number
-Shape
-Surrounding skin (redness/edema/eczema/scars/hyper or hypopigmentation)
-Margin (healed/inflammed/fibrosed)
-Base (granulation tissue/slough)
-Edge (sloping/punched/undermined/rolled/everted)
-Discharge (serous/sanguinous/serosanguinous/purulent)
-Structures visible (muscles/vessels/bone)

PALPATION
-Temperature
-Tenderness
-Edge (soft/firm/hard)
-Floor (bleed to touch/profusely/hemorrhagic spots)
-Base (consistency, underlying structures)
-Fixity (skin/muscle)

REGIONAL LYMPH NODES

DISTAL NEUROVASCULAR STATUS
JOINT MOVEMENTS

THANKS
HELP PATIENT DRESS
WASH HANDS
SUMMARY
DD

VARICOSE VEINS EXAMINATION (PERIPHERAL VENOUS EXAMINATION)

GRADES OF CHRONIC VENOUS DISEASE
-C0s (heavy legs/pains in legs/pruritis but no clinical signs of venous disease)
-C1 (telangiectasia/reticular veins)
-C2 (visible and palpable varicose veins)
-C3 (venous edema without skin changes)
-C4 (skin changes like hemosiderin pigmentation/venous eczema/lipodermatosclerosis/atrophie blanche)
-C5 (healed ulcer with skin changes)
-C6 (active ulcer with skin changes)

(WINCER)
WASH HANDS
INTRODUCTION
NOTICE (check patient details)
CONSENT
EXPOSURE
-to underwear while maintaining dignity
REPOSITION
-initially standing

GENERAL
-look around bed for walking aids/medication/compression stockings

INSPECTION
Inspect from all sides -kneel infront of patient and behind and ask him to turn around
6 S
-site of varicose veins (above SPJ relate to LSV while those below SPJ relate to LSV or SSV) and saphina varix
-skin (venous eczema/hemosiderin deposition/lipodermatosclerosis/hair loss/redness in superficial thrombophlebitis/shiny skin) note gaiter area
-atrophie blanche (white patches found in areas of healed ulceration)
-edema (due to DVT or lymphedema)
-ulcers (medial malleolus for LSV/lateral malleolus for SSV/marjolin's ulcer/periostitis tibia)
BEDS
-scars (groin crease scar/popliteal fossa scar/avulsion scars: small scars along leg in distribution of long and short saphenous veins) from previous varicose surgery
-loss of hair/brittleness of nails (impending gangrene)
-phlegmasia alba dolens (white leg)
-phlegmasia cerulea dolens (cyanotic mottled skin)
-equinus deformity

PALPATION (TT SEC FFP TR)

Ask about pain

Examine good limb first

-temperature

-saphina varix

    -feel at saphenofemoral junction 4cm below and lateral to pubic tubercle

    -cough test (morrisey's cough impulse) (palpate at saphenofemoral junction while patient coughs)

    -palpable thrill

    -tap test (schwartz test) retrograde impulse is felt due to incompetence of valves in GSV (testing for retrograde and orthograde transmission of percussed pulse i.e palpate varicosities and tap below and then above)

-feel down the leg over course of LSV and SSV for tenderness along the veins (perforator incompitence)

-brodie trendelenberg test for SFJ incompetence (SFJ occlude with finger) vs perforator incompetence

- three or multiple tourniquets test for SFJ incompitence and level of incompetence (perforator incompitence)

    -just below SFJ (adductor canal perforator incompetence) dodd

    -just below midthigh (below knee perforator incompetence) boyd

    -just below knee (lower leg perforators incompetence) cocket

-modified perthes test, once tourniquet test has controlled the superficial system, to assess patency of deep venous system (DVT). Ask pt to tip toe or walk will result in engorged varicosities and bursting pain

-pratt's test

-fegan's test

-hand held DOPPLER ASSESSMENT at 45° to skin for SFJ and SPJ (swoosh as you release calf muscle) to hear forward and backward whoosh suggesting incompetence on compressing calf

FOR DVT

-homan's sign (forcible dorsiflexion)

-moses sign (squeezing calf from side to side)

AUSCULTATION

-bruits (femoral arteries/AVF due to post-femoral catheterization or IVDU)

Both limb diameters above and below any fixed bony point to mention any swelling

REGIONAL LYMPH NODES

ARTERIAL SYSTEM

ABDOMINAL EXAMINATION AND DRE

to see any mass

SCROTAL EXAMINATION for varicocele

ABPI

THANKS

HELP PATIENT DRESS

WASH HANDS

SUMMARY

- FBC
- ESR
- CRP
- COAGULATION PROFILE
- GROUP AND SAVE
- LFT
- U&E
- CXR
- ECG
- VENOUS DUPLEX
- VENOGRAM
- HAND HELD DOPPLER
- USG ABDOMEN AND PELVIS